Healthy Skin Plain and Simple

Peggy J. Sanders, Cosmetic Chemist for the personal care industry for 30years.

iUniverse, Inc.
New York   Bloomington

Editing by Katrina A. Thomas and Ron Flesch

Contents

Introduction

The way to have beautiful skin is to generate healthy skin. And that's what this book is all about. It describes what skin is, what it needs and ways to satisfy those needs. It is a guide to the types of products and ingredients available to help you achieve those aims.

To this end there are chapters on the physiology of skin, daily care, sun care, antioxidants, and aging. Scattered throughout are insights into some specific skin problems as well as chapters devoted entirely to psoriasis and acne.

In the back is a glossary of terms to help with those not-so-common words and a dictionary of ingredients as you will find them on product labels.

All in mind to help you focus on your special needs and to more easily wade through the myriad of products in the market to find what you need and want to achieve the goal of healthy beautiful skin.

Skin—What it is

We all care how our skin looks. We want it to be smooth and free of wrinkles and blemishes. But skin is more than a vehicle to beauty. It has many functions: it protects us and regulates our temperature.

"The skin acts as a stretchable protective shield that prevents harmful microorganisms and foreign material from entering the body and prevents the loss of body fluids."[1]

"When sweat is excreted through the pores and then evaporates from the surface of the skin, a cooling effect occurs. On very humid days you are not cooled easily because the outside air is almost saturated with water and sweat merely builds on your skin instead of evaporating. On cold days your skin acts as a sheet of insulation that helps retain body heat and keep your body warm."[2]

Human skin tissue is approximately 90% collagen protein and contains 18–20% of the body water. [3] The fat produced in the sebaceous glands for the skin's surface is called sebum.

The collagen protein is comprised of amino acids. Acids are neutralized by alkaline materials. Weak ones, like amino acids, can be damaged by strong alkaline materials. So it's a good idea to avoid skin contact with those. The usual culprits are hair depilatories, oven cleaners, ammonia and bar soaps.

Water and oil are always present in healthy skin tissue and work together to keep the skin soft and subtle. Water can be lost through

---

1) "Human Anatomy and Physiology," 3rd Edition, Donna Van Wynberghe, Charles R. Novack, and Robert Carola, McGraw-Hill, Inc. New York, New York 1995. p. 136. Printed with permission of McGraw-Hill Companies.

evaporation and that is one reason for the sebum, to prevent water loss. Its other function is to provide lubricity to the skin. How much sebum one's skin produces is determined by your genes.

Also the production of sebum decreases with age. [4] Outside influences such as: dry climate, wind, sun, use of harsh chemicals, depilatory creams, waterless hand cleaners and detergents may exhaust the skin of needed oils as well as water.

On the other end, some genetically produce too much sebum, and in particular production increases with adolescence. Too much may result in blemishes or acne from clogged pores at any age.

Since the water is part of the body's water and evaporation is one way to lose it, it follows that drinking ample amounts of water benefits both the body and the skin.

Replenishing oil and water to the outer layer with lotions and creams also helps to keep the skin healthy.

"The cells in the stratum corneum (outer layer) are constantly being shed through normal abrasion."[5] When you exfoliate the skin these are the cells you are removing.

The outer layer of skin tissue, the epidermis, lies on top of the dermis beneath which lies the connective tissue.

It is through "food routes" in the dermis that the epidermis is nourished. It is here in these tissues that skin aging takes place. These "food routes" become atrophied starving the outside layer.[6] "Wrinkling happens when the protein elastin in the elastic tissue of the dermis loses its resiliency and degenerates into elacin. This causes the dermis to become closely bound to the underlying tissue."[7]

The rate at which one's skin ages depends upon heredity [8] and the respect with which one regards the true meaning of a tan. For the sun which gives us a healthy glow ironically contributes greatly to skin aging. (See section on Sun Care.)

2)   Op. Cit. p.137.

3)   Lecture Notes on Dermatology, Bethel Solomons, Blackwell
     Scientific Publications, London, Oxford, Edinburgh,
     Melbourne, 1948 p.9.

4)   Ibid p.9.

5)   Wynsberghe—Op.Cit. p.133.

6)   Solomon p.9.

7)   Wynsberghe–Op cit. p.137.

8)   Solmon p.9

Cleaning the Skin

Keeping the skin clean is important for two reasons. It keeps the pores from clogging and provides access for therapeutic applications such as anti-aging and age prevention products as well as acne or psoriasis remedies.

With the pores clear, the heating and cooling system is able to work more efficiently. Also it enables them to keep themselves clean, eliminating blemishes such as blackheads and pimples.

In order for anti-aging, age prevention products, acne and psoriasis medicines to have an effect they must have a direct contact with the skin. Dirt and make-up in the way would lessen their effectiveness.

A thorough cleaning would include removal of any make-up, dirt, environmental pollution, exfoliation of dead skin cells and deep cleaning the pores.

MAKE-UP REMOVERS

Make-up is comprised of fine particles of pigment either dry or dispersed in oil or water-in-oil bases. All of which can easily find their way deep into the pores.

To be an effective make-up remover it must be able to seep into the pores to clean them. The most prominent products used are: cold creams and make-up remover cloths.

Cold creams are the oldest form of make-up removers. They are water-in-oil emulsions. This means that the oil remains on the outside of the water so that the product behaves like an oil. Thus giving them the needed ability to seep into the pores and remove oil and/or pigments. The presence of the water cuts down excessive oiliness while the emulsifiers such as borax/beeswax or stearate soaps behave like cleaners and aid in the removal.

Make-up remover cloths are available as reusable or disposable.

The disposable type usually contain some cleaner which is non-oily but capable of removing oil and deep cleaning the pores such as alcohol, glycerin, or hexylene or propylene glycol. They may contain mild surfactants such as sarcosinates, glucosides or betaines.

Eye make-up removers contain mild surfactants that are non-stinging to the eyes.

Reusable remover cloths are a micro-fiber. The fiber technology works so efficiently they mildly exfoliate. In so doing, they enable the pores to self-clean. They can be washed in the regular laundry and reused.

Liquid Skin Cleansers and Shower Gels

These usually contain gentle surfactants: betaines, isethionates, sarcosinates, sulfosuccinates, or glutamates to name a few. Body cleansers for the shower and bath will likely contain conditioning agents such as: glycerin, guar gum derivatives or polyquaterniums. Their pH is about that of the skin, slightly acidic. These are not only gentler to the skin than bar soaps, they don't produce that pesky scum around the tub and shower.

Soap Bars

One of the oldest cleaning tools is the soap bar. They are a product of neutralizing a fatty acid with an alkali. This is called saponification.

Whole tallow or cuts from tallow or vegetable oils such as stearic or oleic acids are used. Sodium or potassium hydroxide or TEA are used as the alkaline neutralizers.

In order to produce a good hard bar the final pH of the soap must be 8 or above, leaving excess alkali in the bar. And these are strong alkalies. This is the downside of soap bars for cleansing. These alkalies will attack the amino acids in the skin's protein causing irritation, dryness or even blemishes. If the skin is inherently oily this might not be a problem. But if the skin is dry it probably will be.

Much of the soap bar does not dissolve in water and instead complexes with minerals in hard water to produce that scum around the sinks, tubs and showers.

SYNDET BARS

Not all cleansing bars are soaps as described above. They can be a combination of surfactants and emollients and are called syndet bars. The surfactants add foam, cleansing and water solubility. They can have a lower pH than that of soaps and can be much gentler to the skin.

FACE MASKS AND SCRUBS

These Products deep clean the pores, exfoliate and tighten the skin.

Masks tighten and dry, pulling water from the pores bringing dirt, oil, and make-up with it. The dead skin cells are removed during the rinse off. Clays, flours, glycerin, synthetic polymers, botanical extracts and celluloses are used as drying agents, tighteners and exfoliants.

Sheet type masks have a variety of purposes. They can soothe or relax as well as tighten and exfoliate. The sheets are treated with botanical extracts to tighten or soothe and/or fruits acids to exfoliate.

Cleaning strips are a variation of masks. They contain cellulose gums, glycerin, titanium dioxide, or clays to tighten and extract dirt and blackheads from the pores.

Scrubs for the face contain mild abrasives such as ground fruit seeds or nuts, bamboo, luffa, finely ground pumice, calcium carbonate, magnesium oxide or polyethylene beads and sometimes a clay to scrub away dead skin cells. They may also contain mild surfactants for sudsing and wetting or even an emollient ingredient.

For the body bath scrub items such as luffa sponges, nylon sponges or microfiber cloths work very well. Pumice stones are excellent for callous removal from elbows, feet or hands.

All of these products unclog the pores allowing them to cleanse themselves properly.

SKIN ASTRINGENT/FRESHENER PRODUCTS

A skin astringent product contracts or shrinks the pores. It has good oil removal capacity for ridding the skin of residual cold cream and or make-up or sebum. It may be used as part of a facial or alone between facials for a quick light refreshing.

Skin astringent products may contain: ethyl (grain) alcohol or isopropyl alcohol, or any of many plant extracts with natural astringent properties; agrimony, alfalfa, basil, black walnut, burdock root, camphor, eucalyptus, grapefruit, chamomile, orange oil, rosemary, sage, thyme, witch hazel, or yarrow.

The alcohol or plant extract cleans the skin as described and may leave behind a cooling effect, due to quick evaporation. This latter property also aids in shrinking the pores. There is another theory that the pores are constricted by inflaming the tissue around them, causing swelling thereby seeming to shrink the pores. But cooling is a verified method of shrinking them and cold water can act as well for this need.

Moisturizing the Skin

Water and oils are always present in the skin. They work together to keep the skin soft, pliable and prevent cracking and irritation.

We lose our natural sebum through cleansing, environmental influences, harsh detergents, cleansers or aging. Without sufficient sebum to occlude evaporation, water can be lost.

Moisturizer products are so named because they not only restore oils and water to the skin they retain moisture there as well. A good one is a light oil in water emulsion with a nongreasy feeling and a true moisturizer contains a humectant. Humectants are any materials that not only hold onto water but pull it from the air as well. Below is a list of humectants:

Acetamide MEA
Dipotassium Glycyrrihizate
Fructose and other sugars
Fructose Oligosaccharides
Glycerin
Glycyrrhetinic Acid
Isostearyl Lactate
Methyl Gluceth 10, (and) 20
Oligosaccharides
Polysaccharides
Amino Acids (hydrolyzed proteins):
Arginine
Glycine
Serine
Proline
Cysteine

Sodium Behenoyl Lactylate
Sodium Isostearyl Lactylate
Sodium Lactate
Sodium Lauroyl Lactylate
Sodium PCA
Sodium Polyasparate
Sodium Stearoy Lactylate
Sorbitol

In addition to humectants there are materials found naturally in the skin called ceramides. These are greatly responsible for the skin's ability to retain its own moisture. It has also been determined that the presence of ceramides diminish with age. Using products containing ceramides at therapeutic levels can restore the skin's ability to hold its water.

Also there is a family of materials made from glutamic acid (an amino acid), and either phytosterol or chloresterol which behave like ceramides. [1] They are by name:

Cholesteryl/behenyl/octyldodecyl/lauroyl glutamate

Cholesteryl/octyldodecyl/lauroyl glutamate

Phytosteryl/behenyl/octyldodecyl/lauroyl glutamate

Phytosteryl/octyldodecyl/lauroyl glutamate

The newest member of this family is based on B-alanine and phytosterol, namely Phytosterol/Decyltetradecyl Myristoyl Methyl Beta-Alaninate and tests show it to have five times the moisture retaining effect of its previous siblings. [2]

1) Ajinimoto

2) Ajinimoto

Sun Care for the Skin

We all enjoy fun in the sun. Many of us play sports like tennis and golf under the glow of the sun. It perks up one's spirits, especially when we haven't seen it for a while due to rain or clouds. The sun is necessary to grow plants and dry out the atmosphere and us.

We need the sun to manufacture Vitamin D. "The skin helps screen out harmful excessive UV rays from the sun, but it also lets in some necessary UV rays, which convert a chemical in the skin called 7-dehydrocholesterol into Vitamin D³ (cholecalciferol)". [1] Also psoriasis sufferers find help from monitored sun exposure.

For various reasons we all need the sun in moderation. But there is danger to the skin from overexposure. It can result in skin cancers and premature aging.

Victims of skin cancer share a history of either long exposure to the sun over a period of years or acute overexposure on an occasional basis. The fairer the skin the less exposure needed to incur damage. Also those living in sunny climates experience a higher incidence of skin cancer. The combination of fair skin living in sunny climates poses the greatest risk and calls for more protection.

The sun's harmful rays also speed up the aging of the skin. [2] To bear this out compare the parts of the body that are continually exposed like the arms, neck, face and legs to the rest of the body that rarely see the sun. What has been said with respect to sun bathing and skin types and skin cancer also applies to skin aging.

When it comes to sun protection, SPF numbers are a good place to start. But it doesn't end there. SPF means Sun Protection Factor. The number indicates how much longer you can stay in the sun without getting burned wearing this product than you could without it. In other words it defines protection from the burning or UVB rays only.

UVB rays penetrate the epidermis but go no further. They cause burning and redness and are a potential cause of skin cancer. "UVB significantly decreases the enzymic and non-enzymic antioxidants in the skin, thus impairing its ability to protect itself against free radicals generated by exposure to sunlight. It is considered to be a potential cause for skin cancer due to DNA damage."[3]

But it has been found that the tanning or UVA rays are longer and penetrate deeper into the dermis. There they do damage to the elastin and collagen in the connective tissue causing premature aging. [4] (see section on Skin-What it is). Their damage is subtle and doesn't show up for years.

That is why we have sunburns to let us know right away that we are overexposing ourselves. If you're protected by a good SPF you're not getting burned and don't realize the damage that you are doing. This is almost worse than no protection. Just because you turned off the alarm doesn't mean that you don't have to get up and go to work.

"Ultraviolet rays also stimulate the melanocytes to produce melanin." "The tanned skin helps to prevent further ultraviolet damage by absorbing and scattering the harmful rays." [5] It is the body's own protection system. Those who have more melanocytes will tan better and have more protection than those who have less and this is determined by hereditary factors. While having a tan protects the skin the process of getting a tan also the damages the skin as mentioned above.

And UVA rays penetrate the ozone layer, window glass and clouds. [6] This last is evidenced by indoor/outdoor glasses which darken even when it's overcast.

There are many ingredients that are effective against the burning rays:

Octylmethoxycinnimate

Octisalate (Octyl Salicylate)

Homosalate (Homomenthyl Salicylate)

Padimate O (Octyl Dimethyl PABA)

Octocrylene

It's protection against the tanning rays that require more careful reading.

Oxybenzone (Benzophenone-3)

Avobenzone (Butyl Methoxydibenzoyl Methane)

Are among those effective against the UVA (tanning) rays. Of these only the latter, avobenzone, is effective against the entire UVA spectrum. [7]

Ingredients such as zinc oxide, and titanium dioxide are physical blocks and are effective against both UVB and UVA rays. They are inorganic materials and as such have the advantage of being chemically stable in sunlight.

Covering with clothing is probably one of the best protection options. It is both economical and practical. The clothing should be made of tightly woven fabrics. Long sleeved t-shirts, light weight trousers, and wide brimmed hats are recommended. Whites and lighter colors reflect the rays while black and darker ones absorb them. In the hot weather whites and pastels would be more comfortable.

If you're planning on spending a long day in the sun you might want to go with the clothing option. If that seems too uncomfortable and you opt for a sunscreen product, it should be reapplied at intervals even if the SPF is high and the product contains avobenzone. These materials can degrade in the sun over time. Plus these products can get worn off by towels and perspiration in spite of water proofing.

Despite planning there will always be times when you find yourself unexpectedly overexposed. There are first aid remedies which can help with that. But they should be employed as soon as possible.

First take a long cool shower to dissipate the heat. Next apply aloe vera which is legendary for its ability to alleviate the pain of burn and its effects. When possible use the undiluted juice from the plant. Next apply an antioxidant. They are quite common, readily available and can prevent damage done by overexposure to the sun.

Remember to be conscious of how much you are exposing yourself to the sun, take necessary precautions when needed. And in case of accidental overexposure apply the first aid measure mentioned above.

Love the sun but always respect it.

1)   Donna Van Wynsberghe, Charles R. Noback, and Robert Carola, "Human Anatomy and Physiology" McGraw-Hill, Inc. New York, Third Edition 1995 p. 137.

2)   Bethel Solomons "Lecture Notes on Dermatology" Blackwell Scientific Publication 1948 p.9.

3)   DSM   Nutritional   Products–(Roche)   "Sun   Exposure, Photoaging and the Protective Anti-aging Effects of Parsol 1789 2nd Edition 1996 p.4.

4)   Ibid p.5.

5)   Wynsberghe p. 139.

6)   DSM p.3.

7)   Ibid p.8.

Antioxidants

Antioxidants help control free radicals and prevent tissue damage. To understand how this works it is necessary to understand what a free radical is and how it behaves.

So we'll go back for a little chemistry 101.

There are 92 natural elements occurring as atoms. All of them, save the six inert gases have an imbalance between the positively charged protons in the nucleus and the negatively charged electrons in the outer shells. They are always striving for a balance. They accomplish this by finding another atom willing to share one or more of its electrons. This bonding satisfies the balance needed and the result is called a molecule.

Usually these bonds are not broken. But when they are this could result in an unstable molecule which is called a free radical. Hydroxyls, superoxides and peroxides are three known free radicals.

This free radical will strive to balance itself by "stealing" an electron from the nearest molecule. This "vicitimized" molecule now becomes a free radical and "steals" an electron from another molecule setting up a chain reaction. In the body this can end in the destruction of a cell or cell DNA.

Antioxidants or oxygen quenchers as they are sometimes called are molecules which can give or share an electron without becoming a free radical itself.

We have many of them in nature:

Vitamin E
Vitamin C
Phytic Acid

Others are:

Alpha Lopoic Acid (Thiotic Acid)
Lutein
Ethylbisiminomethylguaiacol Manganese Chloride

In addition many plant extracts contain antioxidants:

Astaxanthin
Calendula
Centella Asiatic
Coffee Arabiea
Chlorogenic Acid
Date
Echinacea
Ellargic Acid
Ginger Powder
Ginko Biloba
Glycyrrhiza Glabra (Licorice)
Grapeseed
Green Tea
Hawthorne
Jojoba Oil
Kakadu Plum
Pine Bark
Pomegranate
Rooibus Tea (Red Tea)
Terminalia Arjuna Bark
White Tea
Applied topically in lotions, creams or masks, they can deter cell degeneration of the skin. Remember that antioxidants may only prevent damage, they cannot reverse it.

<u>*Preventing Skin Aging*</u>

Nobody wants lines and wrinkles but we all get them anyway. It's only a question of how many, how fast.

Mostly this is determined by hereditary factors over which we have no control. Other than that we can take steps to delay them. As already mentioned protecting from damaging sun rays helps as do antioxidants.(See section on Sun Care).

In addition the industry has been recently blessed with some new tools to prevent aging.

One is an extract from the root of the Oenothera Biennis plant. It works by inhibiting one of the enzymes that damages collagen at the same time it is stimulating collagen synthesis. And since this enzyme is stimulated by the sun, you could say it helps prevent sun damage. [1]

Another age prevention tool is Tripeptide-2. It inhibits other enzymes which damage collagen and elastin. These enzymes are stimulated by the sun as well as environmental factors. [2]

A third tool is Acetyl Hexapeptide-1, which behaves similar to a hormone which stimulates melanocytes to produce melanin. It produces a bit of glow in the skin. Maybe it's like getting a tan without incurring the cellular damage which accompanies it. [3]

These ingredients may be available in skin care products. But their presence there does not guarantee results; they must be present at therapeutic levels. As with all ingredients it isn't just what is in a product but how much.

1)   Soliance

2)   Atrium

3)   Atrium

Reducing Signs of Aging

Once you get the wrinkles help is as close and as simple as a neighborhood drug store for topically applied products. Or if you prefer upper scale products you can make a trip to a spa or a department store.

To Reduce the Appearance of Fine Lines and Wrinkles AHA and Retin A creams are available.

All of these work similarly and the mechanism is simple. AHA stands for Alpha Hydroxy Acid which includes glycolic and other fruit acids. Retin A used to be vitamin A (retinol) that has oxidized to retinoic acid.

The acids chew off the outer layer of the skin causing irritation, plumping the skin thus reducing the appearance of the wrinkles.

Results are visible within 5–10 days.

The effects are not permanent. The cream must be used daily to maintain them. If the products are formulated properly there should be no irritation to the skin in general.

Peels are self-descriptive. They peel off the outer layer of skin cells revealing a fresh layer. Very simply fruit acids are used to do this, chosen for their mildness. They may be thickened with gums to make them easier to handle and apply. After the specified time the product is rinsed from the face leaving behind a new skin layer with more even skin tones and less fine wrinkles and blemishes.

There are more extensive skin peels available at the dermatologist.

<u>Deeper Lines and Wrinkles</u> can be minimized by applying products with combinations of peptides and super moisture retention ingredients.

Polypeptides (oligopeptides, tripeptides, tetrapeptides) aid in collagen and elastin synthesis which is essential to skin tone and elasticity.

The ability of the skin to retain its own moisture plays a big part in keeping the skin plump and fresh looking. As we age we lost some of that. The ingredients which can restore that are the ceramides and the amino acid derivatives discussed in the section on moisturizing.

Polyssacharides and oligossacharides have intense moisture retention attributes which help to plump the skin.

Depending on the combination of ingredients and at what level they are present in a product, results could be visible in one week to two months.

To reduce wrinkles on the forehead and around the eyes there is an ingredient that acts like Botox but is much safer and less painful.

So because it is topically applied as opposed to being injected with a dangerous toxin. (See section on Botox). It relaxes the muscles so that they can't contract reducing the appearance of wrinkles. [1] Its name is <u>Acetyl Hexapeptide-3</u> and is available in creams sold over the counter.

1)   Lipotec/Center Chem, Inc.

Deeper Treatment

Beyond the drug and department stores we can go deeper at the dermatologist.

<u>Microdermabrasion, Chemical Peels, IPL Photo facial treatments and Lazer Resurfacing</u> are all procedures which involve removing the outer layer of the epidermis.

Microdermabrasion is a technique in which tiny crystals are sprayed and mild abrasion is applied. Aluminum or magnesium oxide crystals may be used. This is usually followed by a vacuuming to remove the dead skin cells.

There will be some discomfort and recovery time accompanied by the need for creams and lotions.

Chemical Peels treat a variety of skin imperfections from age spots and freckles to lines and wrinkles. They are among many services offered by The New Age Cosmetic Surgery and Spa in Coronado, CA.

And here is what they have to say about them:

Light peels yield subtle improvements. They make your skin look younger and more vibrant. They may require a few visits with each one taking about an hour. There is no downtime. That is you can return to your regular activities right away.

Medium peels remove more layers. Fine lines, wrinkles and age spots are diminished. They require two or more visits and require one to two days of recovery.

Deep peels produce more dramatic results. The skin is more improved, wrinkles and fine lines are noticeably gone or greatly reduced. And these peels can treat precancerous growths.

This procedure is done once, and recovery can take a few weeks to two months.

It is extremely important to protect your skin with sunscreen after having chemical peels. Following your physicians post-peel instructions will help your skin heal more quickly and reduce possible post-treatment complications.

Which peel is best for you depends upon age, condition of skin and desired results. And this is best determined by a consultation with your doctor.

New Image Cosmetic Surgery and Spa also offers <u>IPL Photo facial</u> treatment. This procedure exposes a broad spectrum of light to the skin's lower layers, promoting new collagen and connective tissue production. This creates new structure and support to the upper skin layer creating a smoother surface and a more youthful appearance.

Some people say that the pulsed light feels like the snap of a rubber band against the skin. While no anesthesia is required, topical creams can be applied for patients who would like that option.

IPL Photo facials slough off dead skin, treat fine lines and wrinkles, effects of rosacea, sun spots and broken capillaries.

The sessions take about 30 minutes and there is no down time. Five to eight sessions will be needed to complete the treatment usually about three weeks apart. The skin continues to improve over time.

<u>A Microlaserpeel</u> is the latest advancement in skin resurfacing and is also offered by New Image Cosmetic Surgery and Spa.

This is performed using an Erbium Laser Peel which is now recognized as a preferred method in skin resurfacing because it combines the best features of the Erbium and Co2 laser procedures, while eliminating the drawbacks of each.

And the physician is able to program a specific plan for each patient. A series of three treatments, two to four weeks apart is usually recommended to treat sun damage.

This procedure removes 50 microns of aged and sun-damaged tissue and in so doing can treat wrinkles, acne scars, skin laxity, keratoses and pigmentary problems with limited downtime.

Recovery time is seven to ten days depending on the areas. The face usually takes seven days while the neck and chest can take ten to fourteen days. Again sunscreens are recommended during this period.

Collagen is boosted in three to four weeks following treatment.

Depending on your individual needs this treatment may need to be repeated every six months.

For more information about chemical peels, IPL Photo facials and Microlaserpeels call:

New Image Cosmetic Surgery and Spa
619-437-1388
Or go to their web site:
www.sandiegolipo.com

BOTOX

For wrinkles around the forehead and eyes, there is Botox treatment which is injections of a weak solution of Botulinum Toxin type A.

In its full strength it causes death by paralyzing respiratory muscles. It is this attribute which freezes the targeted muscles, reducing contractions thereby reducing the appearance of wrinkles. It also reduces your ability to make facial expressions such as smiling and frowning.

Besides the pain and risk the other downside is the expense. As this procedure costs about $300.00 per injection and lasts only about three to four months.

A fairly new injectable for plumping out the wrinkles is made up of micro particles of poly-L-lactic acid. Two or three of these sessions over a few months can last up to two years. [1]

Should you opt for any of these dermatologist procedures it is important that you discuss them thoroughly with your doctor. But before you do that make sure that your doctor is certified by the American Board of Medical Specialties. In some states any doctor with a medical license can call him or herself a cosmetic or plastic surgeon.

To qualify for the board's certification the doctor must have five to seven years of post graduate medical training which includes a general surgery program of three years. They must also pass written and oral tests. [2]

Your best source for referrals and information is the <u>Cosmetic Surgery Information Center.</u> It is a non-profit public benefit organization which provides education and assistance to the public.

Before they recommend a surgeon they will have checked out their history in the community, board certifications, training and experience of their staff, accreditation of their facilities and their history for any disciplinary action against them. They can be reached at 800-535-0380. And their services are free to the public.

(1) Technology Drives the Skin Care Category—M. Fishman—HAPPI-July 2006 p. 30.

(2) Cosmetic Surgery Information Center

Acne

Acne is a condition which results from an excessive production of sebum. Usually occurring during teen years when the production is at its peak. But it can crop up at any age.

A lot of sebum together with dead skin cells and/or dirt clog the pores resulting in white or black heads. These can become infected with bacteria and develop into a pimple.

The remedy is to exfoliate the dead skin cells, reduce the oil, and fight the infection.

Exfoliation should be done gently so as not the scratch the sores and cause scarring. Clay masks and micro fiber cloths are possibilities. Facial cleansers with soft scrubs such as polyethylene beads, bamboo shoots, or luffas make good choices. Avoid products containing pumice or other sharp abrasives such as ground seeds or shells.

Clay masks not only exfoliate but the clay will help dry up the excess oils. Micro fiber clothes do an excellent job of gently removing oils and dirt from the pores.

Many anti-acne products contain salicylic acid and or alcohol to help keep the oil down.

Infection has been fought with antibiotics in the past. But recent research has shown that the bacteria are becoming drug resistant. We will likely see a return to the use of benzoyl peroxide, still a very effective combatant against these bacteria. [1]

Vitamin C and extracts containing vitamin C can be of help used externally. Rooibus or red tea is not only high in vitamin C but contains antioxidants and minerals as well. Acerola or barbados cherry is another good source of natural vitamin C and also contains vitamins B1, B6 and folic acid.

Depending on the severity it may be necessary to contact a physician.

A few common sense tips are: Don't put your hands on your face or pick at the zits. There are bacteria under the fingernails which will increase the likelihood of infection plus it may cause scarring.

Also keep in mind that not all skin outbreaks are acne. It could be the result of very dry skin, allergies, or a reaction to an ingredient in a product.

1)   Dermatology Nursing—April 2004 Vol. 16 No. 2 East Holly Avenue Box 56, Pitman NJ 08071-0056, page 185

Warts

Warts are benign tumors caused by a virus. They appear as a raised area of the skin with pitted and uneven surfaces and are usually the same color as the skin.

They disappear in time but you might want to remove them sooner if they are unsightly. And those on the bottom of the feet, called plantar warts can cause discomfort.

They can be removed with over-the-counter products containing salicylic acid. The other option is to see a doctor.

Psoraisis

Psoriasis is a skin condition that affects as many as 7.5 million Americans, according to the National Institutes of Health. It's not just a skin problem and something that should send you to the dermatologist.

The cause is not known for sure but researchers believe it to be related to the immune system and is genetic. The immune system is miscued and causes the growth of too many skin cells too fast. These cells accumulate on the skin's top layers resulting in scaly lesions.

There is no known cure. It is a lifelong condition requiring lifelong treatment. Psoriasis can become worse and at other times may go into remission. As a systemic disease, symptoms may not always be visible but someone who has psoriasis will always have psoriasis.

There are five kinds of psoriasis: plaque, guttate, inverse, pustular and erythrodermic.

Plaque psoriasis, the most common form comprises about 80% of all cases. It shows up as red inflamed lesions covered by a silvery white scale. It occurs typically on the elbows, knees, scalp and lower back.

Guttate psoriasis manifests itself in small, red individual spots, usually on the trunk or limbs. It most often begins in childhood or early adulthood.

This form may come on quite suddenly and can be brought on by a variety of outside influences. Upper respiratory infections, tonsillitis stress with strep throat is the most common trigger.

Inverse psoriasis is found in skin folds such as under the arms, the groin, the genitals, the buttock and under the breasts. The lesions are very red and lack the scale that plaque psoriasis has.

Pustular psoriasis is white pustules surrounded by red skin. The pus is white blood cells and is not contagious. It usually occurs in adults and is fairly rare.

Erythodermic is a rare form and the skin is intensely red looking like a bad sunburn.

The treatments for psoriasis range from the topical applications to systemic treatments, depending on if the disease is localized (in small areas) or widespread (covering large areas of the body.)

Mild cases can be treated with moisturizers to relieve dryness and itching. Bath solutions containing apple cider vinegar, dead sea salts, Epsom salts or certain oatmeal products can remove scales and soothe the skin. Salicylic acid can help loosen scales so other medicines can penetrate the skin.

More intense cases will need help from the doctor for prescription medicines. These include: Donovex (Vitmamin D-3), steroids, and Tazorac (derived from vitamin A).

For severe cases there are prescription systemic drugs either in the form of a pill or injections. These require a doctor's monitoring as they affect other parts of the body.

Phototherapy which uses UVA and UVB rays is also helpful.

Those with psoriasis may also develop psoriasis arthritic. It results in pain, stiffness and swelling around the joints usually of the hand, wrists, knees, and lower back.

If psoriasis is suspected a trip to a good dermatologist is recommended to get started on the right treatment.

My thanks to the National Psoriasis Foundation who provided this information. They are located at 6600 SW 92th Ave. Ste 300 Portland,Or. 97223-7195. For more information or support go to www.psoriasis.org or call 800-723-9166.

Dictionary

The following dictionary lists ingredients found in skin care products. Ingredients are listed on labels in order beginning with the one of the greatest amount first and so on. Many have benefits but be advised that a therapeutic amount must be present in order for the finished products to have that specific benefit.

A

Acerola Extract–(malpghia punicifolia)–A natural source of vitamin C. From the cherry tree indigenous to the West Indies. Used at the right levels it can help protect skin from damage due to sun rays or it can lighten skin color.

Acetylated Lanolin—A derivative of lanolin used for its emollient properties and as an emulsifier.

Acetyl Cysteine—(N-Acetyl-L-Cysteine)—An amino acid that is a part of the collagen protein.

Acetyl Glutamyl Heptapeptide—It may reduce the appearance of aging when present at the right levels.

Acetyl Hexapeptide-1—It activates the melanin production giving the skin a healthy glow. It can provide some of the protection of a tan without the damage. [1]

31

Acetyl Hexapeptide-3—Used at the right levels it reduces the appearance of lines and wrinkles by relaxing the face muscles similar to Botox injections. (See section on Wrinkles—Reduction of). [2]

Acetyl Tetrapeptide-2—Derived from the youth hormone Thymopoietin it boosts the skin's own defenses and helps regenerate the epidermis. [3]

Acetyl Tetrapeptide-5—Reduces puffiness around the eye area.

Acetyl Tetrapeptide-9—A synthetic polypeptide which has been clinically shown to firm and plump the skin, reducing the appearance of lines and wrinkles. [4]

Acetyl Tyrosine—Aids in sunless tanning products.

Acrylamidopropyltrimonium Chloride/Acrylamide Copolymer— Skin conditioning polymer.

Acrylates Copolymer—A thickener for liquid products such as bath gels.

Agrimony Extract—A plant derived ingredient with astringent properties.

Alanine—Amino acid that is part of collagen protein.

Alfalfa Extract—A plant derived ingredient with astringent properties.

Algae—(also Rouge [red] and Brune [brown] or Ahn Feltia Concinna Extract)—Contains proteins, sugars, and vitamins. Used at the right levels in skin care products it lends a protective film providing moisturization and may promote cell regeneration.

Allantoin—This ingredient has a long history of use in skin care products for its healing ability of acne, seborrhea and skin ulcers. It can give temporary relief to minor skin irritations such as scrapes and windburn.

Almond Butter and Almond Oil—(Prunus Amygdalus Ducis)—The oils and butters expressed from almonds and used in skin care for emollience.

Aloe Barbadensis—(Aloe Vera)—The juice or powder derived from the Aloe Vera plant. The name aloe comes from an Arabic word "alloeh" meaning "bitter and shiny substance". Aloe Vera has a three centuries old history of use in healing wounds which includes the soothing and healing of burns. Though there are no clinical tests to verify it there are reports that it can prevent scarring if used during wound healing.

Aloe Vera—See Aloe Barbadensis.

Alpha Lipoic Acid—thiotic acid—This compound is an antioxidant.

Alteromonas Ferment Extract—This helps to reduce skin irritation caused by shaving and environmental factors.

Aluminum Oxide—Inorganic crystals that may be used in the microdermabrasion process.

Aluminum Starch Octenylsuccinate—A naturally derived polymer used in powder make-ups. Also may be used as a co-emulsifier.

Aluminum Zirchonium Tetrachlorohydrox—A drying agent used in antiperspirants.

Amazonia Nut Oil—Used in skin care for its emollience.

Amazonian White Clay—A naturally occurring mineral it is used in face masks to help remove toxins from the skin while pulling dirt from the pores.

Andographis Paniculato Extract—Taken from the leaves of the plant this extract has a history of use in treating skin disorders and inflammations.

Annato Oil—An oil with a high content of carotenoids which can enhance sun screening.

Apricot Kernel Oil—A natural light oil used for emollience in lotions and creams.

Apricot Seed Powder—Ground seeds used in scrub products.

Arbutin Extract—(Bearberry)—Taken from the leaves of the plant, it has tyrosinase inhibiting attributes which can help to lighten skin color.

Argnine—(L-Arginine)—An amino acid that is part of the collagen protein.

Ascorbic Acid—Vitamin C—An important factor in the formation of collagen. It can help protect the skin against UV radiation with continued topical application. [5]

Ascorbyl Dipalmitate—A material with skin lightening and antioxidant attributes.

Ascorbyl Palmitate—A material with skin lightening and antioxidant attributes.

Asparatic Acid (L-Aspartic Acid)—An amino acid that is part of the collagen protein.

Astaxanthin Extract—It contains antioxidants and can level out skin tones, freckles and age spots.

Australian Myrtle Oil—This oil has antimicrobial properties.

Australian Sandalwood Oil—An oil with antimicrobial and anti-inflammatory properties.

Avocado Oil—A light oil used in lotions and creams for emollience.

Avobenzone—See Butylmethoxydibenzoylmethane. (Parsol 1789).

Azelaic Acid—A material with antibacterial attributes.

1) Atrium

2)   Lipotec/Center Chem

3)   Atrium

4)   Laboratorie Serobiologigues—Div of Cognis France

5)   DSM Nutritional Products Inc. (Roche)—The Ingredients for Success In Cosmetics. Second Edition p.12.

B

Babassu Oil—See Orbignya Okifera Oil.

Bamboo—(Bambusa Arundinaceae)—A plant ground into a powder which is used as an exfollient in scrub products.

Basil Extract—A plant derived ingredient with astringent properties.

Beeswax—Derived from honeycomb bee hives. It is used with sodium borate as an emulsifier in lotions and make-up removers where it also serves an additional function as an aid in cleaning.

Behenyl Alcohol—A heavy fat naturally derived and used for emollience.

Behenylamidopropyl Dimethylamine Behenate—An emollient emulsifier used in lotions and creams.

Behenyl Behenate—A heavy ester with emollient properties.

Benzoic Acid—A fungicide used in personal care products to protect them from mold growth.

Benzoyl Peroxide—An ingredient with a long history of treating acne with good results.

Benzophenone-3—An ingredient that is effective against part of the UVA (tanning) spectrum.

Benzyl Alcohol—A material effective against and used to protect products from bacteria growth.

Benzyl Nicotinate–Stimulates circulation.

Bergamont—A relaxing aromatherapy oil.

Beta Glucan—A good source of this material is Oatmeal. It is a natural co-polymer of glucose. As an immune stimulant and film former it has the ability to soothe dry irritated skin. It can increase collagen synthesis and cell renewal, reducing appearance of fine lines and wrinkle.

Bisabolol—An oil with anti-inflammatory, antioxidant, and antibacterial attributes. Both natural and synthetic are available. The natural being derived from the candeia tree which grows in Brazil.

Black Currant Oil—A light oil derived from the berry and used for its emollient properties.

Black Walnut Extract—A plant derived ingredient with astringent properties.

Borage Seed Oil—A natural ingredient—It is rich in essential fatty acids which are beneficial in preventing moisture loss from the skin. It is used to alleviate inflammatory conditions such as eczema and dermatitis. Also has use in lotions, creams, balms and lip products for its emollience.

Borax—A natural mineral used with beeswax to emulsify and thicken cold creams and make-up removers.

Boron Nitride—An inorganic material derived from Borax. It provides smoothness and a soft feel.

Boswellia Serrata Extract—While it contains antioxidants it is known more for its traditional use in treating skin inflammatory conditions.

Brassoca Campetris/Aleurites Frodi Oil Copolymer—A polymer derived from vegetable oils which forms a film which keeps moisture in creams and lotions. Conversely it resists wear and water rinse off of sunscreen products.

2-Bromo-2-Nitropropane-1,3,Diol—A bacteriastat used to protect products from bacteria growth. Rarely in use now.

Brazil Nut Oil—A natural oil used for emollience.

Burdock Root Extract—A plant derived ingredient with astringent properties.

Butyl Carbomate—A preservative used in products to prevent bacteria growth.

Butylene Glycol—An emollient ingredient used in skin care products to provide smoothness and lubricity.

Butyl Methoxydibenzoylmethane—Avobenzone—Parsol 1789— An ingredient that is effective against the entire UVA (tanning) spectrum.

Butyloctyl Behenate—A vegetable derived emollient ester.

Butyl Cetearate—A vegetable derived emollient ester.

Butyl Stearate—An emollient ester.

Butylparaben—A fungicide used in personal care products to prevent mold growth.

Butyrosperum Parkii—Shea Butter—A butter with great emollience which contains vitamin E. It melts at skin temperature and used in creams, lotions and lip products. It is derived from a tree which grows only in the African Savannah region.

C

Calcium Carbonate—It has a use in bath scrubs for gentle exfoliating.

Calcium Hydroxide—An alkaline material used in hair depilatories for its ability to attack the amino acids in hair to aid in its removal.

Calcium Silicate—An inorganic material with sebum absorbing attributes.

Calcium Stearoyl Lactylate—An emollient emulsifier for creams and lotions.

Calendula Extract—Calendula Officinalis Flower Extract—Marigold extract—contains antioxidants.

Camphor—From the camphor tree—It is a counter irritant for pain, itching and also has astringent properties.

Canadian Willow Herb Extract—Belonging to the evening primrose family, it has a history of use in the treatment of burns. Used mostly as an anti-irritant.

Candelilla Wax—A wax derived from a vegetable source that is used in candles and lip products.

Cannabis Sativa Seed Oil—Hemp Oil—An oil with a dry emollience.

Canola Oil—Derived from corn and used for its emollience in creams and lotions. A favorite in lip balms for its flavor.

Caprooyl Tetrapeptide-3—This material has been shown in tests that it "boosted the production of collagen VII, laminin-5 and fibronectin." This reduces the appearance of lines and wrinkles. [1]

Caprylic/Capric Triglyceride—A light emollient ester with a wide use in lotions and creams.

Capryloyl Glycin—A material with antimicrobial attributes and used for "preservative free" products.

Carbomer—A synthetic material used to thicken water to make gel type products. In lotions and creams it is used as a thickener and emulsion stabilizer.

Carnauba Wax—See Copernica Cerifera.

Castor Oil—See Ricinus Communis Seed Oil.

Castor Maleate—An emollient ester used in body washes.

Centella Asiatic Extract—Used as an anti-inflammatory and it also contains antioxidants.

Ceramides—A natural component of the skin which plays a significant role in the skin's ability to retain moisture. (See Moisturizing the Skin).

Ceresin Wax—A wax comprised of saturated and unsaturated hydrocarbons.

Cetearyl Alcohol—A solid white flake, it is a combination of cetyl and stearyl alcohols. Used for emollience and thickening in creams and lotions.

Ceteareth 10 and 20—Both ingredients have emollient attributes. Either may be used to solubilize fragrances or oils.

Ceteth-10,-15 and-20—These are modified fatty alcohols which are used mostly as co-emulsifiers.

Cetyl Alcohol—A solid white flake. A fatty alcohol used for its emollience and thickening in creams and lotions. It is present in animal fats and vegetable oils. Most of what is used in personal care products is derived from palm oil.

Cetyl Babassuate—An emollient ester derived from a vegetable source.

Cetyl Dimethicone—A silicone used for emollience.

Cetyl Ethylhexanoate—A non-comedogenic emollient ester, used in make-ups and skin care products.

Cetyl Lactate—An emollient ester.

Cetyl Octanoate—Emollient ester used in creams and lotions.

Cetyl Palmitate—An emollient ester used in creams and lotions.

Cetyl Phosphate—An ingredient used to adjust pH and/or to emulsify.

Cetyl Ricinoleate—An emollient ester for creams and lotions.

Chamomile Extract—Known for its soothing and anti-septic properties. Used in skin toning and astringent products.

Chamomile Oil—A relaxing aromatherapy oil.

Chitosan—An ingredient derived from shrimp shells. It forms a film which prevents water loss from the skin.

Chlorogenic Acid—It helps in skin lightening and contains antioxidants.

Cholesteryl/Behenyl/Octyldodecyl Lauroyl Glutamate—Derived from amno acids, alcohols and cholesterol, this material functions like a ceramide. It improves the skin's ability to retain moisture. Tests have shown this ingredient to be effective in repairing damaged skin. [2]

Cholesteryl/Octyldodecyl/Lauroyl Glutamate—Similar to its sister above it is derived from amino acids, alcohols and cholesterol. It functions like a ceramide, improving the skin's own ability to retain moisture. [3]

Citrus Tachibana Peel Extract—Lightens pigmentation such as freckles and spots caused by UV exposure. In Japan it is the traditional orange plant. In Chinese herb medicine the peel is known as "Kippi".

Cocamide DEA—A surfactant derived from coconut oil. It is used in skin cleansers.

Cocamide MEA—A surfactant derived from coconut oil and used in skin cleansers.

Cocamidopropyl Betaine—A gentle surfactant used in hair shampoos and skin cleansers. It is derived from coconut oil.

Cocoa Butter—A butter expressed from the seed kernels of the fruit of the cocoa tree. Used for its emollience.

Cocoglucoside—A mild surfactant used in skin cleansers.

Coconut Oil—Cocos Lucifer—An all purpose oil used for its emollience in creams and lotions. It is also a source of raw materials for many surfactants.

Cocyl Caprylate/Caprate—An emollient ester.

Coffee Arabic Extract—Coffee Bean Extract—Contains powerful antioxidants.

Collagen—This is the protein of which skin is comprised and is used for skin repair.

Coleus Forskohlii Oil—This material has antimicrobial properties and may help combat acne.

Coleus Forskohlii Root Extract—It is used in the treatment of psoriasis.

Copaiba Oil—An oil with a pleasant balsam odor which contains beta-carophylene which provides germicidal action.

Copernica Coperica—Carnauba Wax—A wax scraped from the leaves of the plant belonging to the palm family. It is used in lipsticks as well as candles.

Cucumber Extract—A material which aids in skin lightening.

Cupuacu Butter—A butter which is beneficial to dry skin due to its emollient properties.

Cyclomethicone—A silicone which is volatile and helps to provide a dry after feel.

Cyclopentasiloxane—A silicone which lends a dry feel to a product.

Cysteine—(L-Cysteine)—An amino acid that is a part of the collagen protein.

Cysteine HCl—An amino acid that is a part of the collagen protein.

1)   Atrium

2)   Ajinimoto

3)   Ajinimoto

D

Date Extract—A fruit extract which contains antioxidants and a natural antimicrobial.

Decyl Glucoside—A mild surfactant.

Decyl Oleate—An emollient ester which may be used in place of mineral oil.

Decyltetradecyl Cetearate—An emollient ester derived from vegetable sources.

Devil's Claw—See Harpagophytum Procumens Extract.

Diazolidinyl Urea—A bacteratstat used to protect cosmetic and personal care products from bacteria growth.

Dibehenyl Fumarate—An emollient ester.

Di-^{C12}–^{15} Alkyl Fumarate—An emollient ester which melts at body temperature.

Dicapryl Adipate—An emollient ester with a dry non-oily feel.

Dicapryl Maleate—A noncomedogenic emollient ester.

Dicaprylyl/Capryl Sebacate—An emollient ester derived from castor and palm oils.

Diethyl Hexyl Fumarate—An emollient ester with a dry feel.

Diethyl Hexyl Sebacate—A noncomedogenic emollient ester with a non-greasy feel. Used in make-ups as well as creams and lotions.

Diisodecyl Adipate—An emollient ester with a dry after feel. Also is used to solubilize fragrances in water/alcohol fragrance products.

Diisopropyl Adipate—A noncomedogenic emollient ester with a very light after feel.

Diisopropyl Dimer Dilinoleate—An emollient ester.

Diisostearyl Adipate—A heavy emollient ester.

Diisostearyl Malate—A heavy emollient ester.

Diglyceryl Isostearate—An emollient ester.

Dilauryl Citrate—A co-emulsifier.

Dimethicone—A silicone fluid used in creams and lotions for shine and lubricity.

Dimethicone Copolyol—A silicone surfactant used in skin cleansers for a soft emollient foam.

Dimethicone/Vinyl Dimethicone Cross Polymer—A silicone used in skin care products.

Dimethylcyclopentasiloxane—A silicone fluid used in skin care to add a dryer feel.

Dioctyldodecyl Adipate—An emollient ester.

Dioctyldodecyl Dimer Dilinoleate—A heavy emollient ester, has a feel similar to mineral oil.

Dioctyldodecyl Dodecanedioate—A heavy emollient ester.

Dipalmitoyl Hydroxyproline—Reduces free radicals and may also firm the skin.

Dipotassium Glycyrrhizate—A humectant.

Dipropylene Glycol—Used in skin care products for its emollient attributes.

Disodium Cocamido MEA Sulfosuccinate—A mild surfactant good for face cleansers and eye make-up removers.

Disodium Cocoyl Glutamate—Derived from amino acids this surfactant is very mild to the skin and gentle around the eyes.

Disodium Lauroyl Glutamate—A surfactant derived from amino acids. Mild on the skin and around the eyes.

Disodium Lauryl Sulfosuccinate—A mild surfactant derived from amino acids.

Disteareth-75-PNI—A thickener used in bath gels derived from stearyl alcohol.

Disteareth-100 IPDI—A thickener used in bath gels derived from stearyl alcohol.

Ditridecyl Adipate—A noncomedogenic emollient ester with a dry after feel. Used in lotions, creams and sun care products.

Dodecylhexyldecyl Palmitate—An emollient ester derived from vegetable sources.

DMDM Hydantoin—A bacteriastat used to prevent bacteria growth in personal care products.

E

Echinacea—Contains antioxidants.

EDTA—A chelating agent. It also serves as a preservative booster.

Emu Oil—It has a history of use in Australia in alleviating eczema, psoriasis, burns and dry skin. Used in creams and lotions for its emollient properties.

Elastin—A component of the dermis and used in skin care products for help in skin repair.

Ellagic Acid—An antioxidant, it helps with lightening skin color.

Ethoxydiglycol—An ingredient used to solubilize fragrances and sunscreens.

Ethyl Alcohol—Derived from grain, it is used in astringent products and make-up removers and colognes.

Ethyl Ascorbic Acid—It has the ability to lighten skin color and has antioxidant attributes.

Ethylbisiminomethylguaiacol Manganese Chloride—A powerful antioxidant.

Ethylhexyl Palmitate—An emollient ester for use in creams and lotions.

Ethylhexyl Pelargonate—An emollient ester with a dry, non-oily feel.

Ethylhexyl Salicylate—Octyl Salicylate—Octisalate—An ingredient which is effective against the UVB (burning rays).

Ethylparaben—A fungicide used to prevent mold growth in personal care products.

Erythulose—A natural sugar which produces a natural looking tan by reacting with primary and secondary amino groups to form a brown substance called Melanodin.

Eucalyptus Globulus Leaf Oil—From the leaf of the tree, it contains eucalyptol which has decongestant attributes. It has a history of treating fever, cough and asthma, thus the nickname "Australian fever tree". In skin care it is used for its astringent properties.

Evening Primrose Extract—Whitens the skin by inhibiting tyrosinase activity and the production of melanin.

Evening Primrose Oil—An oil rich in essential fatty acids, containing 74% linoleic acid and 8–10% gamma linolenic acid which are helpful in preventing moisture loss from the skin.

F

Fermental Grape Extract—White Mulberry—It inhibits tyrosinase activity thereby lightening skin color.

Ferula Feotida Root Extract—It evens out skin tones.

Ficus Caria Extract—Fig Extract.

Fig Extract—Fruit extract having natural antimicrobial attributes and containing alpha-hydroxy and malic acids.

Flax Seed Oil—A light lubricious oil.

Fructose Oligossacharides—Humectants with intense moisture retention properties which help to soothe the skin and smooth the cutaneous layer. In addition they contain some beta-carotene and ascorbic acid.

G

Galactoarabinan—Wood Gum or Larch Gum—A polysaccharide extracted from the North American Larch tree. It is used in skin care as a film former which occludes water loss from the skin and has tightening attributes.

Galunga Extract—It has antimicrobial properties and may be used in anti-acne products.

Gentian Extract—Mostly used to treat oily skin, diffuse redness and tighten pores.

Geranium Oil—An aromatherapy oil with stimulating effects.

Ginger Powder—Derived from the ginger spice it contains antioxidants.

Gingko Biloba—Used in China for 2000 years in traditional medicine. It contains antioxidants. If present at the right level it can even out skin tones.

Glutamic Acid—(L-Glutamic Acid)—An amino acid which is a component of collagen protein.

Glutamylamidoethyl Imidazole—Derived form glutamic acid. It can boost the skin's natural defenses.

Glycereth-26—An emollient emulsifier.

Glycereth-2-Cocoate—An emollient thickener.

Glycereth-8-Hydroxystearate—An emollient ester.

Glycerin—Derived from palm oil it is a natural humectant widely used for years in a broad spectrum of skin care products ranging from lotions and creams to make-up removers and toners. Its ability to attract water is sometimes used in masks and cleaning strips to dry and tighten.

Glyceryl Behenate—An emollient emulsifier for creams and lotions.

Glyceryl Cocoate—An emollient emulsifier.

Glyceryl Isostearate—An emulsifier used in creams and lotions.

Glyceryl Oleate—An emulsifier for creams and lotions and used in skin cleansers for its emollient properties.

Glyceryl Polyacrylate—A film former for lotions and creams to prevent water loss.

Glyceryl Polymethacrylate—A film former used in skin peels and masks.

Glyceryl Ricinoleate—An emulsifier for creams and lotions.

Glyceryl Stearate—A widely used emulsifier for creams and lotions.

Glyceryl Stearate Citrate—An emulsifier.

Glyceryl Triisostearate—An emulsifier used in creams and lotions.

Glyceryl Tristearate—An emulsifier.

Glycine—The amino acid which comprises the biggest part of the collagen protein.

Glycol Distearate—Used as a pearlizing agent in lotions and in bath gels and other skin cleansers.

Glycolic Acid—An acid used in antiwrinkle creams and exfoliating products. The mechanism in both types of products is the same. It exfoliates by gently removing the outer layer of skin reducing the appearance of wrinkles.

Glycol Stearate—Used as a pearlizing agent in lotions, bath gels and other skin cleansers.

Glycosaminoglycans—A natural component of the skin which inhibits enzymes which damage collagen.

Glycyrrhetinic Acid—A humectant used in creams and lotions.

Glycyrrhiza Glabra Extract—Licorice—Contains antioxidants and aids in the lightening of skin tones by inhibiting melanin production.

Grapefruit Extract—It has astringent properties.

Grapefruit Oil—An aromatherapy oil with refreshing effects.

Grapeseed Extract–It contains antioxidants.

Grapeseed Oil—A light oil, good for leave on oil products such as after bath and massage oils.

Green Tea Extract—An extract containing high levels of antioxidants called polyphenols. All teas contain these antioxidants in the beginning. Black tea is made by a fermentation process which destroys most of them. If the leaves are steamed dried immediately following the harvest the fermentation does not take place keeping the antioxidants intact. That is green tea.

Guar Hydroxypropyl Trimonium Chloride—Derived from a natural source it is a thickener and conditioner used in shampoos and bath and shower gels.

H

Harpagophytum Procumbers Extract—This plant is indigenous to South Africa where it has had a traditional use in relieving pain and fever. It is recognized as an analgesic and anti-inflammatory agent.

Hawthorne Fruit Extract—Contains antioxidants and has antimicrobial attributes.

Hempseed Oil—Hemp Oil—See Cannabis Sativa Seed Oil.

Hexapeptide-1—A peptide with skin firming attributes.

Hexylene Glycol—An emollient ingredient used in skin care lotions and bath gels.

Homomenthyl Salicylate—See Homosalate.

Homosalate—An ingredient which is effective against the UVB (burning) rays.

Hibiscus Flower Extract—Has astringent properties.

Hydrogenated Cottonseed Oil—Used for its emollient properties.

Hydrogenated Lanolin—A modified lanolin for use in lotions and creams.

Hydrogenated Lecithin—Modified lecithin used as an emulsifier in creams and lotions.

Hydrogenated Olive Oil—A derivative of olive oil used for its emollience.

Hydrogenated Palm Glycerides—A solid emollient ingredient used mostly in lipsticks.

Hydrogenated Palm Kernel Glycerides—A solid emollient ingredient used in lipsticks.

Hydrogenated Palm Kernel Oil—Used for its emollience in skin care products.

Hydrogenated Soybean Oil—Used for its emollience.

Hydrogenated Soy Glycerides—Used for its emollience in creams and lotions.

Hydrolyzed Collagen—The amino acids of collagen protein. Can aid in healing the connective tissue.

Hydrolyzed Elastin—The amino acids of elastin. It has moisturizing properties which improve the suppleness of the skin.

Hydrolyzed Milk Protein—The amino acids of milk protein used as a moisturizer.

Hydrolyzed Silk Protein—Amino acids from the silk protein. Used as a moisture binder.

Hydrolyzed Soy Protein—Amino acids from the soy protein and good moisturizers.

Hydrolyzed Wheat Protein—Amino acids from wheat with moisturizing attributes.

Hydroxyethyl Cellulose—Derived from a natural source it is used as a thickener in skin and hair care products.

Hydroxylated Lanolin—A derivative of lanolin it is used for its emollient properties in lotions and creams.

Hydroxylated Lecithin—An emollient emulsifier.

Hydroxymethyl Dioxolanone—A solvent with emollience.

Hydroxyl Proline—An amino acid which is a component of collagen.

Hydroxypropyl Cellulose/Methyl Gluceth—Serves as a barrier to common irritants.

I

Illipe Butter—Shorea Stenoptera Butter—Similar to cocoa butter with long lasting moisturizing effects used in creams, lotions and lipsticks.

Imidazolinyl Urea—A preservative used to prevent bacteria growth in personal care products.

Isobutylparaben—A fungicide used to protect personal care products from yeast and mold growth.

Isocetyl Ethylhexcanoate—An emollient ester with a dry feel.

Isocetyl Palmitate—An emollient ester.

Isocetyl Stearate—An emollient ester.

Isocetyl Stearoyl Stearate—An emollient ester.

Isodecyl Neopentanoate—An emollient ester with a dry after feel. Used in lipsticks as well as creams and lotions.

Isodecyl Oleate—An emollient ester with a dry feel.

Isododecane—An oil used in skin care products for its emollience.

Isohexadecane—An ingredient used for its emollient properties.

Isononyl Isononanoate—An emollient ester.

Isooctyl Caprylate/Caprate—An emollient ester derived from castor and palm oils.

Isopropyl Alcohol—Commonly called rubbing alcohol, it is used in astringent products and make-up removers.

Isopropyl Lauroyl Sarcosinate—An ingredient derived from amino acids with emollient and high moisture retention attributes. Also can boost the effectiveness of Avobenzone (Butyl Methoxydibenzoyl Methane).

Isopropyl Myristate—An emollient ester used in creams and lotions.

Isopropyl Palmitate—An emollient ester used in creams and lotions.

Isostearamido Morpholine Lactate—A conditioner that lends softness to the after feel.

Isostearamidopropyl Morpholine—A conditioning agent used in skin care products.

Isostearate Behenate—An emollient ester that melts at skin temperature and lends a dry after feel.

Isostearyl Isostearate—An emollient ester.

Isostearyl Lactate—A humectant that may also double as an emulsifier.

Isostearyl Neopentanoate—An emollient ester.

Isostearyl Palmitate—An emollient ester with a non-greasy feel. Used in creams and lotion, lip products and other stick products such as deodorants, etc.

Isostearyl Stearoyl Stearate—A noncomedogenic emollient ester used in lotions and creams and also as a pigment binder in make-up products.

Isostearyl Stearate—An emollient ester.

J

Jojoba Oil—Not really an oil but a mixture of wax esters it is harvested from a shrub which grows in the southwestern U.S. It contains natural tocopherols (vitamin E).

Juniper—A calming aromatherapy Oil.

K

Kakadu Plum Extract—The plum contains up to 4% ascorbic acid. One plum is equivalent to ten oranges. It also contains antioxidants.

Kaolin—A natural clay used in masks for tightening, cleansing and exfoliating.

Kigelia Africana Extract—From a tree which is native to Africa. Provides tightening and firming of skin tissue.

Kojic Acid—As a tyrosinase inhibitor it helps lighten skin tones.

Kokum Butter—Garcinia Indica Seed Butter from the kokum tree which is indigenous to India. It has good moisturizing attributes and melts close to skin temperature.

Kukui Nut Oil—Produced by cold pressing the oil from the nut. It has a non-greasy feel.

L

Lanolin—Fat extracted from the wool shorn from sheep. It is soft and greasy and has a long history of use in lotions and creams for its excellent emollience. It is particularly good for dry skin.

Lanolin Alcohol—A fraction of the lanolin. It is used for its emollience in creams and lotions.

Lauramide DEA—A surfactant derived from coconut oil. It is used in the better hair shampoos and skin cleansers.

Laureth-4—A derivative of coconut oil used for its emollient properties.

Laureth-23—A derivative of coconut oil used as an emulsifier.

Lauric Acid—A fatty acid derived from coconut oil and used mostly to make liquid soaps.

Lauroyl Lysine—Derived from the amino acid, L-Lysine, it offers high lubricity and water repellency to make-ups and powders as well as other skin care products.

Lauryl Glucoside—A mild surfactant in skin cleansers.

Lavender Oil—A calming, relaxing aromatherapy oil.

Lecithin—An emollient emulsifier in creams and lotions.

Lemon Tea Tree Oil—It has insect repellency and antimicrobial properties.

Lentium Edodes Extract—Shiitake—A mushroom from the far east. It contains lentinan, a B-glucan which has antimicrobial and antiviral attributes.

Licorice Extract—From anise, it has skin tightening properties and also contains antioxidants.

Lily Root Extract—It has anti-irritation attributes.

Linoleamide DEA—A surfactant made from the unsaturated oils found in vegetable oil mostly safflower oil. It has a smooth soft feel.

Linoleic Acid—An unsaturated fat derived from sunflower, corn, or cottonseed oil.

Linolenic Acid—An unsaturated fat derived from linseed oil.

Locust Bean Gum—Ceratonia Siliqua—A natural gum used in thickening products such as face masks.

Lotus Powder—From the lotus seeds it is used as an exfoliant.

Luffa—A fibrous plant used in scrubs or as a sponge to exfoliate.

Lutein—Belongs to the family of carotenoids, and is an antioxidant found naturally in the body.

M

Macadamia—Brown granules of the ground nut. Used as an exfoliant.

Macadamia Nut Oil—(Ternifolia Seed Oil)—Oil produced by cold pressing of the nut.

Magnesium Aluminum Silicate—Natural clays used in masks for drying and exfoliating.

Magnesium Ascorbic Phosphate—A stable form of vitamin C which is hydrolyzed back to vitamin C by the skin's own enzymes. It can lighten skin tones and promote collagen synthesis.

Magnesium Oxide—Inorganic crystals which may be used in the microdermabrasion process.

Mangifera Indica Leaf Extract—Mango—Contains antioxidants, and has anti-inflammatory attributes.

Mangifera Indica—Mango Butter—The fat expressed from the seed of the mango. A noncomedogenic butter melting at skin temperature. It is used in creams, lotions and lipsticks.

Marigold Extract—See Calendula Extract.

Melaleuca Alternifolia Oil—See Tea Tree Oil.

Melanin—A natural UV protector and antioxidant produced by the melanocytes in the skin. It is the dominant color in Caucasian and darker skinned peoples.

Menthol—An alcohol derived from peppermint oil. It is used for its cooling effect in shaving products.

Menthyl Lactate—It is derived from menthol and has cooling attributes good for shaving and massage products.

Methylcellulose—A gum used to thicken bath and shower gels.

Methylchloroisothiazolinone/Methylisothiazolinone—Always used together to prevent bacteria growth in cosmetics and personal care products.

Methyldibromo Glutaronile—A fungicide used in personal care and cosmetics to prevent molds and yeasts.

Methyl Gluceth-10 and-20—They are both humectants.

Methyl Glucose Dioleate—An emollient emulsifier for lotions and creams.

Methyl Glucose Isostearate—An ester derived from sugar and used as a co-emulsifier.

Methyl Glucose Sesquistearate—An emulsifier.

Methylparaben—A fungicide and bactericide with a 50 year history of use as a preservative in food and personal care products. It is known to be absorbed through the skin and from the gastrointestinal tract. But tests conducted by the Berdock Group on Vero Beach, Florida (Oct. 2002) show that it is hydrolyzed to p-hydroxybenzoic acid, conjugated and rapidly excreted in the urine. There is no evidence of accumulation. And it is not carcinogenic or mutagenic. [1]

Microcrystalline Wax—A wax with a small crystalline structure used in lipsticks, pomades and ointments. It is derived from hydrocarbons.

Mineral Oil—A highly refined oil derived from hydrocarbon sources. It has a long history of use in personal care and baby products, i.e., lotions, make-up removers, moisturizers, and baby oils and lotions.

Morus Alba Extract—Mulberry—It inhibits melanin production helping to even skin tones.

Mowrah Butter—Madhuca Latifola Seed Oil—Obtained from the fruit of the tree. It melts at skin temperature. It has good emollience for creams and lotions.

Murumuru Butter—A fat high in oleic acid, providing much softness and emollience.

Myreth-3-Ethylhexanoate—An emollient ester used in stick deodorants.

Myreth-3 Myristate—An emollient ester for lotions and creams.

Myristamidopropyl PG-dimonium—A conditioner for skin cleansers, also lotions and creams.

Myristyl Lactate—An emollient ester for creams and lotions.

Myristyl Myristate—an emollient ester used in creams.

Myrrh—A soothing aromatherapy oil.

1)   U. S. Department of Labor, OSHA.

N

Neem Oil—Melia Azadirachta Seed Oil—This oil has a traditional use in the healing of skin disorders such as eczema, psoriasis, rashes, burns and acne. Some consider it to be a natural insect repellent.

O

Oat Flour—Made from oats, it is used to thicken and add softness.

Oat Meal—A source of beta-glucan. (see).

Octisalate—See Ethylhexyl Salicylate.

Octocrylene—An ingredient which is effective against the UVB (burning) rays and is water proof.

Octyl Dimethyl PABA—Padimate O—An ingredient which is effective against the UVB rays.

Octyldodecyl Isostearate—An emollient ester.

Octyldodecyl Myristate—An emollient ester.

Octyldodecyl Neopentanoate—An emollient ester with a dry feel.

Octyldodecyl Stearate—An emollient ester.

Octyl Hydroxy Stearate—An emollient ester.

Octyl Isononanoate—An emollient ester with a dry after feel.

Octyldodecyl Stearoy Stearate—An ester used mostly as a pigment disperser in make-ups and a binder in pressed powders.

Octylmethoxy Cinnimate—An ingredient which is effective against the burning rays.

Octyl Palmitate—An emollient ester with soft dry feel similar to that of the oil on a duck's feathers.

Octyl Salicylate—See Ethylhexyl Salicylate.

Oenothera biennis—An extract from the root of the plant. It inhibits enzyme activity which damages collagen and simultaneously stimulates collagen synthesis. [1]

Olea Europaea Butter—Produced from cold pressing the olive. It has a feel similar to shea butter. It is good for body massage creams.

Olea Europaea Fruit Oil—Olive Oil—Expressed from the olive fruit with a high content (78%) of oleic acid. This oil has a traditional use of relieving stings and burns.

Oleic Acid—A fatty acid derived from olive oil. It is used mostly to make soaps, in particular clear glycerin soaps.

Oleth-2,-5,-10 and-20—Derivatives of olive oil used as emulsifiers or to solubilize fragrances and oils.

Oleyl Betaine—An amphoteric surfactant with a luxurious feel used mostly in bath and shower gels.

Oligosaccharides—An ingredient with long lasting moisturizing attributes.

Olive Extract—A natural antimicrobial with moisturizing attributes and contains antioxidants as well.

Olive Oil—See Olea Europaea Fruit Oil.

Olive Oil PEG-7 Esters—Ingredients used in skin care derived form olive oil.

Orange Oil—It is used for its astringent properties.

Orange Powder—It is made from the peel of the fruit and used as an exfoliant.

Orbignya Oleifera Seed Oil—Babassu Oil—Basbassu is a palm tree indigenous to Brazil. The oil melts at skin temperature, and used in creams, lotions, and lipsticks.

Oxybenzone—See Benozphenone-3.

Ozokerite Wax—Wax derived from a hydrocarbon source, used in various stick products.

1)   Soliance

P

Padimate O—See Octyl Dimethyl PABA

Palmitoyl Dipeptide—An ingredient that may be helpful in wound healing.

Palmitoyl Hexapeptide-6—If present at the right levels it can stimulate collagen synthesis reducing the appearance of wrinkles.

Palmitoyl Oligopeptide—If present at the right levels it has the ability to stimulate collagen synthesis, firming the skin, reducing the appearance of wrinkles.

Palmitoyl Tetrapeptide-3—By stimulating collagen synthesis it plumps the skin reducing the appearance of wrinkles.

Palmitoyl Tripeptide-3—If present at the right levels it has the ability to stimulate collagen synthesis, firming the skin, reducing the appearance of wrinkles.

Palmitoyl Tripeptide-8—It can soothe dermatis, eczema and rosacea conditions and provide relief after dermatological procedures such as microdermabrasion, lazer treatments and chemical peels.[1]

Panthenol—A precursor to pantothenic acid, vitamin B^5, which is present in all living cells. There are d-(dex) panthenol and dl-panthenols. For skin care d-panthenol works best providing penetrating moisturizing and possibly aids in tissue repair. For nails its deep penetrating moisturization protects against breakage. In hair products dl-panthenol is best. It penetrates the hair shaft where it becomes pantothenic acid restoring resiliency and preventing breakage.

Papaya—An extract rich in polysaccharides which are moisturizers.

Paraffin Wax—A synthetic wax made from hydrocarbons, used in stick products such as lipsticks and balms.

Paraguay Tea Extract—An extract with tightening attributes.

Passion Flower Oil—A relaxing aromatherapy oil.

Passion Fruit Oil—An oil used for its emollient attributes.

PEG-14 Butyl Ether—Used for emollience.

PEG-6 Caprylic/Capric Glycerides—Used for emollience in bath and shower gels.

PEG-8 Caprylic/Capric Glycerides—Used as an emollient emulsifier.

PEG-40 Castor Oil—A modified castor oil which may be used to solubilize fragrances and oils or as an emulsifier.

PEG-4 Diheptanoate—An emollient ingredient for skin care.

PEG-8 Dimethicone—A water soluble silicone fluid.

PEG-12-Dimethicone—A silicone surfactant with low eye and skin irritation.

PEG-7 Glyceryl Cocoate—A derivative of coconut oil it is used in bath and shower gels for its emollience. It may also sometimes be used as an emulsifier.

PEG-20 and PEG-30 Glyceryl Stearate—They are both emulsifiers.

PEG-7, PEG-30, and PEG-80 Glyceryl Soyate—They are all gentle cleansers for bath and shower gels.

PEG-75 Lanolin—A derivative of lanolin used to solubilize fragrances and oils.

PEG-120 Methyl Glucose Dioleate—An emollient ingredient.

PEG-20 Methyl Glucose Sesquistearate—An emulsifier.

PEG-15 Soyamine/IPDI Copolymer Dimer Dilinoleate—A conditioner used in bath and shower gels.

PEG-40,-50 and-100 Stearate—They are all three emulsifiers.

Pentaerythrityl Distearate—An emollient ester.

Pentaerythrityl Tetrabehenate—An emollient ester for skin care products.

Pentaerythrityl Tetra Ethylhexanoate—A heavy ester which adds a wet feel and imparts lubricity to skin care products.

Pentaerythrityl Tetrastearate—An emollient ester.

Pentapeptide-3—An ingredient which can reduce the appearance of wrinkles by stimulating collagen synthesis.

Peppermint Oil—A stimulating aromatherapy oil.

Petrolatum—A refined soft solid derived from mineral oil, it has a long history of use in lip balms, hot oil treatments, ointments and salves.

Phenoxyethanol—A bacteriastat used to prevent bacteria growth in personal care and cosmetic products.

Phospholipids—These are materials that are very effective in preventing moisture loss from the skin.

Phytantriol—A building block of vitamin E. It is substantive to hair, skin and nails and reduces moisture loss.

Phytosterols—These are emollient ingredients derived from natural sources such as algae. They may also stimulate biological activity of the skin.

Phytosterol/Decyltetradecyl Myristoyl Methyl Beta-alaninate— Amino acid derived ingredient that restores the skin's ability to retain its own moisture. [2]

Phytosteryl/Behenyl/Octyl/Dodecyl/Lauroyl Glutamate— Derived from an amino acid, fatty alcohols and phytosterol it has the ability to restore the skin's own ability to retain moisture. [3]

Phytosteryl/Octyl/Dodecyl/Lauroy/Glutamate—Derived from an amino acid, fatty alcohols and phytosterol it has the ability to restore the skin's own ability to retain moisture.[4]

Pine Bark Extract—An extract containing antioxidants.

Polyacrylamide (and) C^{13-15} Isoparaffin (and) Laureth-7—An ingredient which is used as a thickener and emulsifier for creams and lotions.

Polydodecanamideaminium Triazadiphenyl-ethenesulfonate— A material which emits and diffuses light to diminish the appearance of wrinkles.

Polyethylene—Usually in bead form and used in scrubs and deep pore cleansers for mild exfoliation.

Polyglyceryl-4 Diisostearate—In combination with Polyhydroxystearate/Sebacate it forms an emulsifying system.

Polyglyceryl-4 Laurate—A co-emulsifier.

Polygonum Multiflorum Extract—Taken from the roots of the plant it contains antioxidants and can even out skin tones.

Polyhydroxystearate/Sebacate—See Polyglyceryl-4 Diisostearate.

Polypeptide—This ingredient can stimulate collagen and elastin synthesis, firming the skin and reducing the appearance of wrinkles if present at the right level.

Polyquaterniums 7, 10 and 73—Hair and skin conditioning polymers used in hair and body shampoos.

Polysorbates-20,—60, and-80—They have many uses either as co-emulsifiers or to solubilize fragrances and oils.

Pomegranate Fruit Extract—(Punica granatum)—An extract which contains anthocyanidins which have a very high antioxidant activity surpassing that of red wine, red tea or green tea.

Pomegranate Powder—From the seeds of the pomegranate, it is used in scrubs for gentle exfoliation.

Porphyridum Cruetum Extract—It contains high molecular weight polyssacharides and oligo-metals. It increases the total lipids in the epidermis and if present at the right levels in the product may improve the skin's elasticity.

Potassium Cocoyl Glycinate—A gentle surfactant good for skin cleansers.

Potassium Thioglycolate—A material used in depilatories to break apart the protein structure of hair for easy removal.

Potassium Sorbate—It is used as a fungicide to prevent mold growth in products.

PPG-2 Isoceteth-20 Acetate—An emulsifier in creams and lotions. It may also be used to solubilize fragrances or oils.

PPG-3 Hydrogenated Castor Oil—An emollient ingredient which provides gloss in lipsticks.

PPG-10 (or)-20 Methylglucose Ether—Either ingredient may function as a humectant or to solubilize fragrances or oils.

PPG-20 Methylglucose Ether Distearate—An emollient ester.

PPG-3 Myristyl Ether—An ingredient used for its emollient properties.

PPG-12 PEG-50 Lanolin—A derivative of lanolin.

PPG-15 Stearyl Ether—An emollient ingredient which may be used to solubilize fragrances, oils, etc.

Proline—(L-Proline)—An amino acid which is a component of collagen.

Propylene Glycol—A ingredient used for its emollient properties which also adds smoothness and lubricity to lotions and creams.

Propylene Glycol Caprylate—An emollient ingredient derived from vegetable sources.

Propylene Glycol Ceteth-3 Acetate—A noncomedogenic emollient ingredient used as an emulsifier or a pigment wetter.

Propylene Glycol Dicaprylate/Disparate—An emollient ester for skin care.

Propylene Glycol Isoceteth-3 Acetate—An emollient emulsifier.

Propylene Glycol Myristyl Ether Acetate—An ingredient with emollience similar to lanolin.

Propylparaben—A fungicide used to prevent mold growth in products.

Prunus Cerasus—Bitter Cherry—It contains a high level of provitamin A (carotenoid).

Pueraria Mirifica Root Extract—An extract which is high in phytoestrogens which can help reduce the appearance of aging.

Pumice—A mineral, derived from lava, used for exfoliating. It is available in stone form for removing calluses from feet and elbows or it may be used in its ground up form in scrubs and masks.

PVP—Film former, moisturizer.

PVP/VA Copolymer—A film former used in peel-off masks.

PVP/Polycarbamyl/Polyglycol Ester—A water resistant film former.

1) Atrium

2) Ajinimoto

3) Ajinimoto

4) Ajinimoto

Q

Quaternium 26—A conditioning polymer for bath and shower gels.

R

Retinoic Acid—Oxidized vitamin A. As a mild acid it is used in anti-wrinkle products. It exfoliates the outer layer of skin resulting in subsequent puffing reducing the appearance of lines.

Retinol—Vitamin A. It is very unstable and rarely used in products for this reason.

Retinyl Palmitate—An ester form of vitamin A, the most stable form of the vitamin and used in products. It is converted to vitamin A by the skin's own enzymes. And vitamin A can increase elasticity, help thicken the epidermis and help dry skin.[1] In anti-wrinkle products it further oxidizes to retinoic acid. (See Retinoic Acid)

Ricinus Commumis Seed Oil—Castor Oil—An oil used for its emollience or as the starting material to make other ingredients.

Rooibus Extract—Red Tea, Redbush or Masai—A member of the camellia sinensis family. It contains a high percentage of antioxidants, vitamin C and minerals. It has been known to relieve sunburn, eczema and acne. It is naturally caffeine free.

Rosemary Oil—An aromatherapy oil with invigorating effects.

Rose Oil—An aromatherapy oil with calming effects.

Rumex Occidentalis Extract—An extract with the ability to tighten skin.

37)   DSM Nutritional Products, Inc. (Roche) The ingredients for Success in Cosmetics p.8.

S

Saccharomyces Ferment Lysate—An ingredient which stimulates production of soluble elastin which may reduce the appearance of wrinkles and sagging skin.

Saccharomces Lysate Extract—It can sooth inflamed skin.

Safflower Oil—A vegetable oil containing about 74% linoleic acid, an unsaturated fat. It is used for emollience.

Sage Extract—An extract with astringent properties.

Salicylic Acid—A mild organic acid used in anti-acne products to help dry up the excess sebum.

Sandalwood—An aphrodisiac aromatherapy oil.

Scieretium Gum—A skin soother and moisturizer.

Scutell area baicalensis Extract—An extract with the ability to even skin tones by inhibiting melanin production.

Serine (L-Serine)—An amino acid that is a part of the collagen protein.

Sesame Oil—An oil expressed from sesame seeds and contains about 40% linoleic and oleic acids each.

Shea Butter—See Butyrosperum Parkii.

Shea Oil—The liguid part of the shea butter.

Shikakae Extract—Acacia concinna—A plant that grows in arid regions and has a natural lather. It has a history of use in the treatment of skin and scalp inflammations.

Shorea Robusta Seed Butter—A butter with good emollience, melting close to skin temperature. Good for lipsticks, balms and creams.

Shorea Steroptera Butter—See Illipe butter.

Silk Worm Extract—An extract with skin tightening properties.

Silkworm Lipids—An oil which occludes water loss from the skin. It contains linolenic and linoleic acids, phytosterols and ceramides.

Sirchin Oil—Jojoba Oil.

Sodium Behenoyl Lactylate—A humectant and an emulsifier.

Sodium Benzoate—A fungicide used to prevent mold growth in products.

Sodium Bicarbonate—An inorganic salt which is used in bath salts. It helps to soften skin.

Sodium Carbonate—An inorganic salt used in bath salts and soaks to soften the water and sooth the skin.

Sodium Cocoapmphoacetate—An amphoteric surfactant noted for its mildness.

Sodium Cocoate—A soap made from sodium hydroxide and fatty acids from coconut oil.

Sodium Cocoyl Alaninate—A mild surfactant for skin washes.

Sodium Cocoyl Glutamate—A mild surfactant derived from amino acid and is used in bath and shower gels.

Sodium Cocoyl Isethionate—A surfactant used mainly in syndet bars.

Sodium Cocoyl Methyl Taurate—A gentle cleanser for skin washes.

Sodium Cocoyl Sarcosinate—An amino acid derived surfactant, very mild to skin and eyes.

Sodium Hexametaphosphate—An inorganic salt used in bath salts and soaks.

Sodium Hyaluronate—A moisturizer that may be obtained from rooster's combs or a vegetable source. It is powerful enough to be effective at very low levels of use.

Sodium Hydroxide—A very strong inorganic alkaline substance. It is combined with fatty acids to make soaps. On rare occasions it is used as a pH adjuster. Also used in hair depilatories for its ability to break apart the protein structure in hair to aid in easy removal.

Sodium Isethionate—A surfactant used in syndet bars.

Sodium Isostearyl Lactylate—A humectant.

Sodium Lauroamphoacetate—An amphoteric surfactant known for its mildness.

Sodium Laurate—A soap made from sodium hydroxide and lauric acid.

Sodium Lauroy Isethionate—A surfactant used in syndet bars.

Sodium Lauroyl Lactylate—A humectant and an emulsifier.

Sodium Lauroyl Sarcosinate—An amino acid based surfactant that is very gentle to skin and eyes.

Sodium Lauryl Sulfoacetate—A mild surfactant good for skin cleansers.

Sodium Magnesium Silicate—A clay used in masks for cleaning and exfoliating.

Sodium Myristyl Sarcosinate—An amino acid based surfactant very mild to skin and eyes.

Sodium Palmitate—A soap made from sodium hydroxide and palmitic acid.

Sodium PCA—A humectant found naturally in the skin. What is used in products is derived from L-glutamic acid.

Sodium PEG-7 Olive Oil Carboxylate—An emollient ingredient derived from olive oil.

Sodium Polyasparate—A humectant derived from an amino acid, aspartic.

Sodium Shale Oil Sulfonate—It has anti-inflammatory attributes making it effective in the relief of itching. It has antimicrobial properties as well making it effective in the treatment of acne.

Sodium Stearoyl Glutamate—An emulsifier.

Sodium Stearoyl Lactylate—A humectant and emulsifier.

Sodium Tallowate—A soap made from sodium hydroxide and tallow.

Sodium Trideceth Sulfate—A surfactant used in skin washes.

Soluble Collagen—An ingredient used as a moisturizer.

Sorbeth-20—An emulsifier.

Sorbitol—A humectant used in skin care products.

Sorbitan Laurate—A co-emulsifier.

Sorbitan Oleate—A co-emulsifier.

Sorbitan Stearate—A co-emulsifier.

Soyamine DEA—A surfactant derived from soy oil which may be used in bath and shower gels.

Soyamidopropyl Betaine—A surfactant derived from soy used in bath and shower gels.

Soybean Oil—An oil used for its emollient properties.

Squalene—An ingredient with excellent emollient properties derived from either shark liver or vegetable sources.

Steareth-2—An emulsifier.

Stearic Acid—A fatty acid which can be derived from either animal or vegetable sources. It is used to make bar soaps like sodium stearate. Or it may be used as an emulsifier in creams and lotions as TEA stearate.

Stearyl Alcohol—A fatty alcohol used in lotions and creams for its emollient properties and its ability to thicken products. While it is available from both animal vegetable sources what is used in personal care and cosmetics is usually vegetable derived.

Stearyl Behenate—An emollient ester.

Stearyl Betaine—A mild surfactant used in skin cleansers.

Stearyl Stearate—A heavy emollient ester for use in lotions and creams and stick products.

Stearyl Stearoyl Stearate—A solid used in stick products for its emollient properties.

Sucrose Distearate, Sucrose Laurate, Sucrose Palmitate and Sucrose Stearate—Emulsifiers derived from sugar and coconut oil.

Sunflower Oil—An oil used in bath oils, lotions, and creams. Derived from sunflower seeds, it contains about 60% linoleic and about 20% oleic acids.

Sunflowerseedamidopropyl Ethyldimonium Ethosulfate—A skin conditioner used in bath and shower gels.

T

Talc—A soft mineral used in bath powders and make-ups.

Tamanu Oil—Bora Bora Oil or Tahiti Oil—Contains calophyllic acid which has regenerating and healing properties. It has a traditional use in the treatment of burns.

TEA—Triethanoamine—A mild alkaline material sometimes used to adjust pH. Most often used with stearic acid to make TEA Stearate to emulsify and thicken lotions and creams and to neutralize carbomers to enable them to thicken and stabilize.

TEA Cocoyl Glutamate—An amino acid derived surfactant, very mild to skin and eyes.

TEA Lauroyl Glutamate—An amino acid derived surfactant, very mild to skin and eyes.

TEA Lauryl Sulfate—A mild surfactant derived from coconut oil.

Tea Tree Oil—An oil with a fresh spicy odor. Due to its antimicrobial properties it is used to treat acne, ringworm, and other sores. It can have a healing effect on blisters, burns and warts.

Terminalia Arjuna Bark Extract—An extract containing antioxidants.

Tetradecyloctadecyl Hexyldecanoate—An emollient ester.

Tetrasodium EDTA—A chelating agent. It is also used as a preservative booster.

Thyme Extract—An extract with astringent properties.

Thyme Oil—An invigorating aromatherapy oil.

Titanium Dioxide—An inorganic ingredient which may be used as a physical sun block in sun care, effective against both UVB and UVA spectra. Or it may be used as a drying agent in skin peels, or as an opacifier in make-ups.

Tocopherol—Vitamin E—A natural antioxidant in the body, its use in personal care products is that of maintaining their stability, safety and purity; and protection of vitamin A derivatives. [1]

Tocopheryl Acetate—Vitamin E Acetate—When topically applied it provides antioxidant protection to the skin. There is also evidence that it soothes and aids in wound healing.[2]

Tribehenin—A heavy emollient ingredient.

Tricapric/caprylic Triglycerides—A light emollient ester used in lotions and creams.

Tricapryl Citrate—A noncomedogenic emollient ester.

Triclocarban—An antimicrobial ingredient used in bar soaps and cleaners.

Triclosan—An antimicrobial ingredient used in hand cleaners.

Tridecyl Behenate—A noncomedogenic emollient ester which liquefies on contact with the skin. Used in creams, lotions and ointments.

Tridecyl Ethylhexanoate—A noncomedogenic emollient ester used in make-ups, lotions, creams and lipsticks.

Tridecyl Neopentanoate—An emollient ester with a dry, non-oily feel. It can be an SFP booster.

Tridecyl Stearate—An emollient ester for skin care products.

Tridecyl Trimelliate—An emollient ester for skin care products.

Triisocetyl Citrate—A noncomedogenic emollient ester.

Triisostearin—An emollient ingredient for creams, lotions and stick products.

Trioctyldodecyl Citrate—A noncomedogenic heavy emollient ester. Its uses are similar to that of castor oil.

Tripeptide-1—If present at the right levels it increases the firmness of the skin by activating the synthesis of collagen and elastin, reducing the appearance of wrinkles.

Tripeptide-2—If present at the right levels it can prevent some skin aging by inhibiting enzyme activity which destroys collagen. At the same time it stimulates collagen synthesis restoring firmness and elasticity to the skin. [3]

Trisodium EDTA—A chelating agent which is also used as a preservative booster.

Triundecanoin—An emollient ingredient used in creams and stick products.

1)   DSM Nutritional Products, Inc. (Roche)—The Ingredients for Success in Cosmetics, p. 6.

2)   DSM Nutritional Products, Inc/(Roche) Ibid p.5.

3)   Atrium

U

Urea—Used as a humectant and disinfectant.

Uva Ursi—Bearberry—An extract which can lighten skin tones by inhibiting the production of melanin.

V

Vanilla Butyl Ether—A warming agent for skin care products.

Vitamin C—See Ascorbic Acid

Vitamin A—See Retinol.

Vitamin A Palmitate—See Retinyl Palmitate.

Vitamin E—See Tocopherol.

Vitamin E Acetate—See Tocopheryl Acetate.

W

Wheat Germ Oil—Triticum Vulgare—Oil from the wheat germ.

White Tea Extract—Contains antioxidants.

Witch Hazel Extract—A fluid extracted from the leaves of the Hamamelis Virginian, a plant indigenous to North America. The extract contains minerals, organic acids, essential oils and tannins. It has a long history of use in skin care for its astringent properties.

X

Xanthan Gum—A natural polysaccharide used as a thickener in lotions, creams, scrubs and masks.

Y

Yarrow Extract—An extract with astringent properties.

Yeast Extract—Reinforces the skin's natural defenses.

Ylang Ylang—An aromatherapy oil with aphrodisiac effects.

Yucca Extract—It is used for its moisturizing properties.

Z

Zanthoxylum Alatum Extract—An extract with soothing properties.

Zinc Oxide—An inorganic material which may be used in sun screen products as a block which is effective against both UVA and UVB rays. Or it may be used as an opacifier in make-ups.

For more information on cosmetic ingredients go to:

www.cosmeticsinfo.org.

Glossary of Terms

Acid—A compound which when dissolved in water gives off H^+ (Hydrogen ions). Many organic acids are mild and non-corrosive such as vinegar. Stearic and Oleic acids are even sometimes used for their emollience. Most inorganic acids are corrosive or irritating to the skin, i.e., hydrochloric or sulfuric. Acids are neutralized with alkalis. One instance of this is the making of soap from stearic acid and sodium hydroxide.

Alkali—An inorganic compound which when dissolved in water gives off OH^-(hydroxyl ions). Sodium hydroxide and potassium hydroxide are examples of harsh alkalis which in their full strength can burn the skin. As a residual in soap they can cause irritation. On the other extreme Sodium Bicarbonate is mild enough to be used as an antacid remedy for the stomach.

Amino Acid–The molecular unit of which all proteins are made. They are present in all living tissue and necessary for tissue repair. There are 20 naturally occurring ones.

Amphoteric Surfactant—Mild cleansing ingredients used in hair and skin washes.

Antimicrobial—Any material which kills bacteria. The same as a bacteriacide.

Aromatherapy—The practice of evoking certain feelings or moods using fragrances.

Astringent—Used to describe an ingredient which draws tissue together or constricts the pores.

Bacteriacide—See antimicrobial.

Bacteriastat—A material which prevents bacteria growth.

Carotene—The yellow pigment in vegetable and animals and the dominant color in Asian skin.

Carotenoids—Yellow to deep red pigment in vegetables and animals. They also stimulate biological activity of the skin.

Carcinogenic—Any material which promotes or causes cancer.

Chelating Agent—Any ingredient which complexes with the minerals in hard water to prevent them from interfering with the cleaning process.

Collagen—The protein present in skin tissue.

Comedogenic—Describes any material which has the ability to cause irritation resulting in skin blemishes or rashes.

Conditioner—An emollient material with a positive charge on one end which enables it to attach itself to the skin or hair lending a soft feel.

Connective Tissue—A skin layer consisting of collagen, elastin and reticular fibers.

Eczema—A chronic irritation of the skin brought on by allergic reactions.

Elastin—A component of the dermis.

Emollient—Having the ability to soften or soothe hair or skin.

Emulsifier—An ingredient in lotions and creams which binds the water and oil phases together.

Emulsion—A homogeneous mixture of water and oil. If there is more water than oil the result is tiny drops of oil in water and called an oil in water emulsion such as: lotions, creams and moisturizers. If there is more oil than water the result is tiny drops of water in oil called a water in oil emulsion such as: balms, ointments and cold creams.

Essential fatty acids—EFA—Long chained polyunsaturated fats which help to reduce moisture loss from the skin.

Ester—An organic compound made from an acid and an alcohol. Many in the beauty business are used for their emollience or as emulsifiers.

Fungicide—A material capable of killing fungus and yeast.

Glycerides—Esters of glycerin and fatty acids or another name for fat.

Humectant—Any substance which holds onto water and pulls it from its surroundings.

Hydrogenation—The process by which hydrogens are added to unsaturated fats making them saturated.

Hydrocarbon—Organic compounds made of hydrogen and carbon usually derived from coal tar or petroleum.

Inorganic—Materials that are not part of living tissue i.e. minerals.

Lipids—Fats.

Melanin—The brown pigment dominant in Caucasian and darker skin coloring.

Melanocytes—The cells in the skin which produce melanin.

Mutagenic—Describes any material capable of causing birth defects.

Non-comedogenic—Describes materials which have been shown not to cause blemishes.

Peptide—An organic compound with amino acids as a part of its chemical structure.

Poly—A prefix meaning many.

Polymer—A very large molecule comprised of smaller molecular units repeatedly linked together in a long chain. Most of what we use is synthetically derived but polymers were first discovered to occur naturally in trees.

Protein—Complex organic molecules made from any of the 20 naturally occurring amino acids.

Rosacea—Acne breakout characterized by redness around the nose and cheeks.

Saturated Fats—Chains of carbons linked to each other by single bonds with the remaining bonds linked to hydrogens. They are very stable. Said to be saturated because the molecule is holding all of the hydrogens it can hold. Examples: stearic acid, stearyl alcohol, cetyl alcohol. A big source of these is palm oil and animal fats.

Surfactant—Any material which lowers or alters the surface tension of water. Some are used in hair and body shampoos to enable water to clean. Others serve as emulsifiers in lotions and creams while yet others solubilize fragrances, oils, etc.

Synergism—The phenomenon of two substances which when used together produce results greater than the sum of the two, i.e., 1+1=4.

Tyrosinase—An enzyme which plays a role in the production of melanin.

Unsaturated Fat—Chains of carbons that are made in an environment where an unsufficient amount of hydrogen is available. The result is carbon atoms forced to bond with each other more than once resulting in double bonds. These are very unstable and easy to break. So called unsaturated because the carbon chain is not holding all the hydrogen it can. Examples: Oleic acid with one double bond found in olive oil; linoleic acid with two double bonds found in safflower oil, cottonseed, and corn oils; linolenic acid with 3 double bonds found mostly in linseed oil.

Bibliography

Ajinimoto USA
West 115 Century Road
Paramus, NJ 07652

Atrium Biotechnologies
1405, boulevard du Parc-Technologigue
Quebec, QC G1P4P5
Canada

Centerchem, Inc.
20 Glover Ave.
Norwalk, CT 06850
(Lipotech)

Cosmetic Surgery Information Center
23175 LaCadena Drive
Laguna Hills, CA 92653

Dermatology Nursing
East Holly Avenue Box 56
Pitman, NJ 08071–0056

DSM Nutritional Products
45 Waterview Blvd.
Parsippany, NJ 07054
Brochures:
The Ingredients for Success In Cosmetics
Sun Exposure, Photoaging and the Protective & Anti-aging
Effects of Parsol 1789

HAPPI—A Rodman Publication
70 Hilltop Road
Ramsey, NJ 07446

Human Anatomy and Physiology 3rd Edition
Donna Van Wynsberghe, Charles R. Noback, Robert Carola
McGraw-Hill, Inc.
New York, New York 1012-2298 1995

Laboratorie Serobiologigues
Division of Cognis France
Ambler, PA

Lecture Notes on Dermatology 4th Edition
Bethel Solomons
Blackwell Scientific Publications
London, Oxford, Edinburgh, Melbourne 1948

National Psosiasis Foundation
6600 SW 92nd Ave. Suite 300
Portland, OR 97223–7195
800-723-9166
www.psoriasis.org

New Image Cosmetic Surgery and Spa
230 Prospect Place Suite 350
Coronado, CA. 92118
619-437-1388
www.sandiegolipo.com

Soliance
30 Place de la Madelaine
75008 Paris
Contact: Paolo Marchesi

U.S. Department of Labor
OSHA
200 Consitution Ave. NW
Washington, DC 20210

www.ingramcontent.com/pod-product-compliance
Lightning Source LLC
Chambersburg PA
CBHW030402290526
45785CB00004B/1863

*9 7 8 0 5 9 5 4 5 3 6 3 4 *